Natural Remedies for Jock Itch
Top 50 Natural Jock Itch Remedies Recipes for Beginners in Quick and Easy Steps

Rita Clark

Copyright © 2015 Rita Clark

All rights reserved.

ISBN-10: 1511687282

ISBN-13: 9781511687287

CONTENTS

Introduction	7
Part 1: Remedies from your Kitchen!	9
Recipe 1: Onion and Aloe Vera paste	10
Recipe 2: Garlic and Olive oil ointment	11
Recipe 3: Honey Garlic Paste	12
Recipe 4: Salt Bath	13
Recipe 5: Apple Cider Vinegar ointment	14
Recipe 6: White Vinegar and Coconut oil therapy	15
Recipe 7: Baking soda bath	16
Recipe 8: Cornstarch remedy	17
Recipe 9: Mustard Seeds Treatment	18
Recipe 10: Turmeric and Honey ointment	19
Recipe 11: Papaya Seed therapy	20
Recipe 12: Yogurt paste	21
Recipe 13: Ice cube cold compress	22
Recipe 14: Fruit peel treatment	23
Recipe 15: Grapefruit Seed extract paste	24
Part 2: Remedies with herbs	25
Recipe 16: Neem paste	26
Recipe 17: Aloe Vera treatment	27
Recipe 18: Chamomile tea therapy	28
Recipe 19: Goldenseal Root therapy	29
Recipe 20: Olive leaf treatment	30
Recipe 21: Lemongrass tea rinse	31
Recipe 22: Basil Leaf paste	32
Recipe 23: Calendula wash	33
Recipe 24: Fig leaf paste	34
Recipe 25: Licorice herbal water rinse	35
Recipe 26: Black Walnut tincture	36
Part 3: Oil Therapies	37
Recipe 27: Tea Tree oil therapy	38
Recipe 28: Coconut oil treatment	39
Recipe 29: Oregano oil therapy	40

Recipe 30: Olive oil and lemon peel therapy	41
Recipe 31: Peppermint oil therapy	42
Recipe 32: Jasmine and orange oil treatment	43
Recipe 33: Lavender oil therapy	44
Recipe 34: Black walnut oil treatment	45
Recipe 35: Wormwood oil application	46
Part 4: Gain immunity with food!	47
Recipe 36: Apple Carrot Pear juice	48
Recipe 37: Tomato delight	49
Recipe 38: Immune boost up Chicken Soup	50
Recipe 39: Immunity building green smoothie	51
Recipe 40: Creamy mushrooms and beans	52
Part 5: Miscellaneous Remedies	53
Recipe 41: Bleach bath	54
Recipe 42: Listerine mouthwash treatment	55
Recipe 43: Alcohol therapy	56
Recipe 44: Nail polish and nail polish remover treatment	57
Recipe 45: Anti-dandruff shampoo therapy	58
Recipe 46: Camphor therapy	59
Recipe 47: Myrrh treatment	60
Recipe 48: Colloidal silver rub	61
Recipe 49: Green clay pack	62
Recipe 50: Petroleum Jelly treatment	63
Conclusion	64
About The Author	66

Introduction

Skin fungal infection is quite common, out of which Jock Itch is a common condition that is caused by a fungus named Tinea. That is why Jock Itch is also known medically as Tinea Crusis. Tinea fungus generally attacks on the moist, warm areas of the body, specifically the genitals, groin area, buttocks and inner thighs. Although it affects both women and men, the high number of infection is observed in men. Obesity, extreme sweating, wearing close-fitting underwear and weak immune system are some of the other causes of Jock Itch.

After reading the above description about this disease, you can imagine how painful it could be. Yes, because Jock Itch is visible as red rashes very much similar to Ringworms. The red patches create great inflammation and itching hence it is really hurting and agonizing. Flaking of the skin also occurs when Jock Itch is at its extreme stage. As per medical experts, Jock Itch is not a serious and life-threatening condition, but it's contagious, therefore needs to be treated well on time.

Though various over the counter medications are available for curing this hurting disease, you can treat it yourself at home using some of the best natural products. Home remedies are successful in treating various diseases without using artificial products and for Jock Itch, such therapies proved extremely beneficial.

However, you need to be a little patient while applying home therapies as they take their own time to heal your skin unlike strong drugs prescribed by doctors.

So, relax and read on the top recipes that we have provided here using naturally safe products for your comfort!

Part 1: Remedies from your Kitchen!

Veggies, fruits and spices that we generally use to prepare meals are loaded with nutrition, but do you know that some of them are extremely beneficial for making home remedial products for curing certain diseases. Yes, common cold and cough and various skin and internal body infections can be treated permanently with our kitchen stuff. So, let's discover some home therapies for curing Jock Itch using kitchen ingredients.

Recipe 1: Onion and Aloe Vera paste

Onion usually brings tears to your eyes when cut, but here onion paste is a great remedy that is able to bring relief in Jock Itch ailment. Onion has anti-inflammatory, antibiotic and antifungal properties that together make it a wonder ingredient to kill the irritating fungus that reasons Jock Itch. Along with Aloe Vera, this paste is really soothing.

Ingredients:

- Onion – 1 medium
- Aloe Vera gel – 2 tablespoons

Method:

Grind onion to a smooth paste. Mix Aloe Vera with the paste and apply it to the affected area. Initially, the onion may give a burning sensation, but it will minimize gradually. Rinse the paste with lukewarm after 30 minutes and clean the area properly. Let the area dry completely. Repeat this process 2-3 times in a day. In a weak or so you will get relief from your ailment.

Variation: Onion oil or onion juice can also be used instead of onion paste

Recipe 2: Garlic and Olive oil ointment

Like the onion, garlic also has antifungal properties, which give immense benefit in treating Jock Itch by restricting growth of fungus on affected area. Here is a nice and advantageous ointment getting relief in Jock Itch.

Ingredients:

- Garlic – 4 cloves
- Olive oil – 2 tablespoons

Method:

In a small pan, take olive oil and fry the garlic cloves. Strain the oil and remove the fried cloves. Now use this ointment in the diseased area for soothing effect. Garlic will kill the fungus whereas olive oil will lubricate the flaked skin. Wash off the ointment after 20-30 minutes. Apply it 3-4 times in a day, especially after taking bath.

Recipe 3: Honey Garlic Paste

Another recipe for Jock Itch remedy with goodness of pure honey and garlic. Honey gives the comforting effect to the itchy and inflammatory area along with its antifungal and antiseptic properties. Garlic with honey is a great combo to give respite from hurting Jock Itch condition.

Ingredients:

- Manuka Honey – 2 teaspoons
- Garlic – 2-3 cloves

Method:

Mince the garlic cloves and mix with honey. Apply this paste to the affected area and leave it for about 30 minutes. Due to garlic, you may feel a little stinging effect, but soon it will vanish. Repeat this application daily once until you get the desired results.

Honey can also be used alone on infected skin twice a day to clear the septicity.

Recipe 4: Salt Bath

This is one of the most inexpensive cure for Jock Itch. You will need table salt for this, but if you have Epsom salt that it would be great. To kill the fungus for clearing the infection and to avoid blisters, this salt bath is excellent.

Method:

In a bathtub full of warm water, add a good amount of salt. Mix well and soak yourself in it for about 20-30 minutes. Let the water touch your infected skin. You can even rub gently your affected area while soaking in water. Take this salt bath twice in a day for better results.

Recipe 5: Apple Cider Vinegar ointment

For all types of skin infections, Apple cider vinegar is quite helpful because of its antibacterial and antifungal properties. This ointment is made using apple cider vinegar and olive oil to give maximum relief from inflammation due to Jock itch.

Ingredients:

- Apple Cider vinegar – 2 tablespoons
- Olive oil – 1 tablespoon
- Warm water – 2 cups

Method:

Combine all ingredients and wash your infected skin with this. Let this solution dry. Do not remove or rub it. Repeat this process 2-3 times in a day for desired results.

Recipe 6: White Vinegar and Coconut oil therapy

Like cider vinegar, white vinegar also has antibacterial and antifungal properties that work best in treatment of skin infections. Now coconut oil we all know is one of the best oils for the skin. So repeat this below therapy 2-3 times in a day and get rid of the Jock Itch infection successfully.

Ingredients:

- White Vinegar – 1 tablespoon
- Coconut oil – 1 tablespoon

Method:

Mix oil and vinegar and apply this solution to your infected area. Let the solution there for 15-20 minutes and rinse it off. Pat dry your skin. After regular use you will see flaky skin that will come out to clear your infectious skin.

Recipe 7: Baking soda bath

Bathing and keeping yourself clean are the top ways to get rid of all types of skin infections and if your bath is treated as a curing treatment then it doubles your chances to clear your infection. Baking soda allows your skin to heal by removing the fungus and the flakes that occur due to infection.

Ingredients:

- Baking soda – ½ cup
- Apple cider vinegar – 2 cups
- Epsom salt – ½ cup

Method:

Mix all these ingredients in your bath tub. Soak in this healing water for about 20-30 minutes. Pat yourself dry, especially the infected area. Repeat this bath twice daily for fast results.

Recipe 8: Cornstarch remedy

Cornstarch is a powdery product made of dried corns. You know that it is the key component in baby powders because of its smoothness and soft texture. This is the reason that experts recommend it for treating Jock Itch where dry skin is necessary for fast healing of infection.

Method:

To soothe your burning sensation occurring in the infected area, apply a little cornstarch on your affected skin. Do it especially when you are going out as chances of perspiration are more when you are moving. Apply it regularly to make your affected area dry as fast as possible. Flakes will come out and the infection will clear out soon.

Recipe 9: Mustard Seeds Treatment

Mustard seeds are said to reduce inflammation and itchiness on the skin so this treatment will be a boon for Jock Itch. It will clear the infection also to offer smooth, healed skin.

Ingredients:

- Mustard seeds – 1 teaspoon
- Water – 1 tablespoon
- Coconut oil – 1 teaspoon

Method:

Soak mustard seeds in water for a while. Grind them into a paste. Now combine the mustard seed paste with coconut oil and apply it over your infected skin. Let it dry for about 45 minutes to one hour. Wash it off and pat dry your skin. Repeat it daily and you will see the good results soon.

Recipe 10: Turmeric and Honey ointment

Honey is soothing while turmeric is antiseptic and both will clear your skin infection with regular application of this ointment. Moreover, your infection will not spread to other parts of your body if you apply turmeric honey paste on the affected area.

Ingredients:

- Turmeric – 2 teaspoons
- Honey – 2 teaspoons

Method:

Combine honey and turmeric. Mix well to make an ointment. Apply over infected area smoothly. It may itch initially, but will give a calming effect later on. Leave it for an hour and wash it off. Repeat the same process thrice a day to get rid of Jock Itch.

Recipe 11: Papaya Seed therapy

Papaya seeds are believed to have therapeutic values that can heal the fungus-infected area with regular usage. Oral consumption is also beneficial while application of seed paste will give relief quickly.

Ingredients:

- Dried Papaya seeds – 1 tablespoon
- Water – little

Method:

Grind papaya seeds to form a powder. Now add little water to make seed paste. Apply this paste to infected skin. Allow it to dry for around 20 minutes and rinse it off. Do this treatment 2-3 times a day to clear the infection permanently.

Variation: You can also rub a piece of fresh raw papaya on your affected area to get calming effect and permanent relief from the infection. Enzymes that are present in Papaya are helpful in killing the infectious fungus.

Recipe 12: Yogurt paste

Yogurt is an antibacterial element containing 'good bacteria' that restrict the growth of infectious bacteria. Doctors recommend regular consumption of yogurt to get relief in skin infections, but for quick results it is good to apply the yogurt paste directly to affected area. Mix it up with honey to make a 'magic' paste.

Ingredients:

- Yogurt – 1 tablespoon
- Honey – 1 tablespoon

Method:

Combine honey and yogurt to make a smooth paste. Apply it on the infected area and let it be there for about 20-25 minutes. Wash it off and pat dry your skin. Repeat this process for twice a day and see the best results!

Recipe 13: Ice cube cold compress

It is the same technique, which your mom applied when you were a kid. Don't you remember the ice cube pack which you mom used to put on your wound to stop itchiness or inflammation? Yes, this the one that you can now apply to your severe Jock Itch infection.

Method:

Place lots of ice cubes in a plastic bag to make the ice pack. Apply that pack on your rashes. Remove the pack in every 2-3 minutes and keep on repeating the process for 10-12 minutes. This will give reduce the inflammation caused due to skin infection and will also let your rashes dry fast.

Recipe 14: Fruit peel treatment

Not only fruits, but some fruit peels also have therapeutic properties that can cure various ailments including skin diseases. Banana, Orange and squash peels are anti-bacterial in nature and can heal your skin very quickly. These peels also contain Vitamin C that is very good in curing Jock Itch

Ingredients:

- Dried peel of 1 orange
- Dried peel of 1 squash
- Honey – ½ teaspoon

Method:

Grind both the peels to form smooth powder. Mix it with honey and make a paste. Apply it on the infected area and leave it on for 20 minutes. Rinse it off with warm water and pat your skin dry. Repeat this treatment twice a day and get instant relief from skin irritation and infection.

Recipe 15: Grapefruit Seed extract paste

This healthy fruit is loaded with Vitamin C that helps in healing rough and infectious skin. Its seeds are also equally therapeutic hence widely used to make skin packs for curing infections.

Ingredients:

- Dried grapefruit seeds – 1 tablespoon
- Honey – 1 teaspoon

Method:

Grind seeds to make powder. Mix with honey and apply the paste to the affected area. Leave it for 20 minutes, then rinse it off. Repeat the same process twice a day and within a few days your infection will get clearer.

Part 2: Remedies with herbs

Herbs like Basil, Neem, Calendula, Olive leaf etc. are believed to have excellent antibacterial and antifungal properties that are essentially needed to heal the Jock Itch infected skin. With these amazing qualities herbs are widely used in making several remedies for curing all types of skin infection. Here also, we have collected a number of remedies in which herbs play a key role in treating Jock Itch permanently without any side effects.

Recipe 16: Neem paste

Neem or Margosa leaves are extremely powerful in healing all types of skin infections by killing the fungus and bacteria present on the skin. It has anti-inflammatory properties as well that make this herb quite excellent in giving a relaxing effect on your rashes.

Ingredients:

- Neem leaves – a handful
- Neem oil – 1 tablespoon
- Water – 1 tablespoon

Method:

Make neem paste by grinding neem leaves, water and oil together. Apply this paste on your infectious skin and leave it for 30 minutes. Wash it off and pat dry your skin. This wonder paste will treat your infections very quick while giving soothing effect on your burning skin.

Recipe 17: Aloe Vera treatment

Aloe Vera has properties that work wonderfully for skin. Whether you have wrinkles or acne or you have severe Jock Itch like condition, regular application of Aloe Vera gel can heal your skin well. Its anti-bacterial elements penetrate deep inside your skin and give you comfort by eliminating bad bacteria.

Ingredients:

- Aloe Vera gel -1 tablespoon
- Olive oil – 1 tablespoon

Method:

Combine gel and oil together. Apply the solution on your rashes and leave it on for 20 minutes. Clean with a moist cotton ball. Repeat it twice a day. You will see your flaky skin and rashes will clean off in a few days.

Recipe 18: Chamomile tea therapy

Chamomile is a great herb, which is widely used as a skin healer. It helps in curing wounds and calming skin irritation and this is the reason that this tea concoction has been recommended for treating Jock Itch condition.

Ingredients:

- Chamomile leaves – 1 teaspoon (Fresh or dried)
- Water – 1 cup

Method:

Boil Chamomile leaves for a few minutes in water. Let all nutrients of the herb come in the water. Strain the water and remove the herbs. Let it cool at room temperature. Dip a cotton ball in the liquid and apply the solution on your rashes. Repeat the process until all liquid is used. Let the area dry on its own. Do this therapy twice a day and you will notice great relief from Jock Itch.

Recipe 19: Goldenseal Root therapy

Goldenseal is an herb that contains antifungal properties in its active compound called Berberine. Due to its medicinal properties it can be consumed in the form of tincture or tablet as well as its root powder can be applied to skin to cure rashes, ringworm or Jock Itch.

Ingredients:

- Goldenseal root powder – 1 teaspoon
- Water – 1 teaspoon

Method:

Combine herb powder with water and make a smooth paste. Apply it on your rashes and leave it on for 20 minutes. Rinse with warm water for clean skin. Do it twice a day for a few days and your skin will be clear of infection.

Recipe 20: Olive leaf treatment

Olive leaf is an antifungal herb obtained from a specific part of the Olive tree. The extract taken from the olive leaf is a highly active component that can treat Jock Itch and other such fungal attacks on the skin. You can either consume this extract to build up your immune system or it can be used as an ointment to clear the skin infection permanently.

Ingredients:

- Olive leaves – a handful
- Water – 1 cup

Method:

Boil olive leaves in water for about 5-7 minutes to extract all nutrients from the leaves. Strain the water and remove the leaves. Now dip a cotton ball in the liquid and apply the solution to your infected skin. Do it until all liquid is finished. Let it dry on its own. Repeat this process of 2 times in a day for a few days. Your infection will disappear real fast.

Recipe 21: Lemongrass tea rinse

Lemongrass tea rinse or compress is one of the best herbal remedies to cure Jock Itch and similar skin infections due to the medicinal properties of Lemongrass. Also, this herb is easily available at herbal stores as well as in grocery shops.

Ingredients:

- Lemongrass – few strands
- Water – 1 cup

Method:

Boil lemongrass in water for a few minutes to extract the medicinal properties of the herb. Dip a cotton ball in the liquid and apply it to your skin on infection. Do it until all solution is used. Let it dry on its own.

Variation: You can even drink lemongrass tea and apply lemongrass oil on affected area.

Recipe 22: Basil Leaf paste

Basil or Holy Basil has great healing and antiseptic properties that can treat various skin problems. In Jock Itch condition, basil leaves prove quite beneficial as a regular application of basil leaf paste can give a soothing effect to your skin.

Ingredients:

- Basil Leaves – handful
- Water – 1 teaspoon
- Coconut oil – 1 teaspoon

Method:

Grind basil leaves with water to make a paste. Mix coconut oil in the paste to make an ointment. Apply it on your infectious skin. Let it be there for 15- 20 minutes. Wash it off with warm water and pat dry your skin. Daily repeat this process for twice a day. In a few days your infection will surely disappear.

Recipe 23: Calendula wash

Calendula is an herb that is best used for beautiful skin due to its antibacterial properties. The leaves of Calendula can be orally ingested in the form of tea for a strong immune system or can be applied externally to heal the skin infections.

Ingredients:

- Calendula leaves – a handful
- Olive oil – 1 teaspoon
- Water – 1 tablespoon

Method:

Grind Calendula leaves with water to make a paste. Mix olive oil with herb paste to form a lotion. Apply this lotion to your infectious skin. Let it be there for 15- 20 minutes. Wash it off with warm water and pat dry your skin. Daily repeat this process for twice a day. In a few days, your infection will clear off.

Recipe 24: Fig leaf paste

Like other herbs, Fig leaf is also said to be a beneficial plant leaf that contains healing properties to treat various skin infections and irritations. However, special precautions should be taken by the people who have sensitive skin. Also, usage of fig leaf juice can make your skin prone to skin burn so avoid prolonged exposure to sun after its application on skin.

Ingredients:

- Fig leaves – a handful
- Water – 1 tablespoon
- Coconut oil – 1 tablespoon

Method:

Make a paste by grinding Fig leaves with water and mix it with coconut oil. Apply this paste to your infectious skin. Let it dry for 15-20 minutes and wash it off. Pat dry your skin.

Recipe 25: Licorice herbal water rinse

Due to its robust antifungal properties, Licorice herb is widely used in making herbal remedies for treating skin fungal infections. For Jock Itch condition, Licorice herbal water rinse is an effective remedy, if it is applied at least thrice or four times a day.

Ingredients:

- Licorice root powder – 7 teaspoons
- Water – 1 cup

Method:

Boil Licorice powder in water for 20 minutes and let it steep for at least 10 minutes. Using a cotton ball, apply this herbal water on infected skin or rinse the area with this water. Repeat this process thrice a day for a few days continuously to get best results.

Recipe 26: Black Walnut tincture

Black Walnut is a widely used herb in Ayurvedic skin therapies. It has a strong healing power due to immense antifungal properties and its oral consumption must be done after proper prescription from expert healer. However, herb tincture can be used externally on skin without any fear.

Ingredients:

- Black walnut herb – a handful
- Water – 1 cup

Method:

Boil herb in water for around 20 minutes and let it steep for 10 minutes to extract its antifungal properties. Using a cotton ball, apply the tincture on affected area and let it dry on its own.

Part 3: Oil Therapies

Herbal oil, natural oil and essential oil; all are extremely good at providing calming effects on the skin. Moreover, if there is any skin infection with high level of burning sensation, these oils prove quite helpful in curing the affected area within a few applications. You can mix these oils with other remedial elements to have a strong and fast effect on your infection. So, read on to know more about these oils and their healing properties. Our home remedies provided below using various oil treatments will let your infection vanish without leaving any mark!

Recipe 27: Tea Tree oil therapy

For effective treatment of Jock Itch, Tea Tree oil is one of the best options due to its strong antibacterial and antifungal properties. It also has stimulating and deep cleansing elements that clear the infection from deep inside the skin. All your irritation and skin inflammation linked with Jock Itch will definitely suppress with Tea Tree oil application.

Ingredients:

- Tea Tree oil – 1 teaspoon
- Coconut oil – 1 tablespoon

Method:

Mix both the oils together. Tea tree oil may cause a little burning sensation on the affected area so to soothe your skin coconut oil is mixed. Using a cotton ball, apply this oil mixture on the infected skin and leave it on for 30 minutes and wash it off with warm water. Pat dry. Repeat this process twice a day for a few days until the infection disappears completely.

Recipe 28: Coconut oil treatment

Coconut oil is well known for its extraordinary healing properties. This is the best oil for skin infections and otherwise also it benefits the skin in many ways.

Ingredients:

- Coconut oil – 1 tablespoon
- Honey – 1 tablespoon

Method:

Mix honey and coconut oil together to form a soothing ointment. Apply it all over your infected area and leave it on for 30 minutes. Let this ointment penetrate into your skin for deep cleansing. Wash off the area and pat dry your skin. Repeat this process twice a day for few days until entire infection vanishes.

Recipe 29: Oregano oil therapy

Containing strong antiseptic compounds like carvacrol, thymol and phenols; this oregano oil is best used as antifungal treatment. However, due to its high potency, it is recommended to use after doctor's advice. Also, it should be used always with some carrier oil to reduce irritation that can be caused after applying Oregano oil on skin.

Ingredients:

- Oregano oil – 1 drop
- Sweet almond oil – 2 tablespoons

Method:

Combine both the oils together to make an ointment. Using a cotton ball, apply it to the affected area and leave it. At regular intervals in a day, apply this oil mixture on your infected skin for best results.

Recipe 30: Olive oil and lemon peel therapy

Olive oil is like coconut oil that can considered 'universal oil'. It is basically a carrier oil that can be used in various home remedies for curing skin infections. Along with lemon peel's Vitamin C properties, this therapy can give maximum relief from Jock Itch infection.

Ingredients:

- Dried lemon peel powder – 1 tablespoon
- Olive oil – 1 tablespoon

Method:

Mix peel powder and olive oil together to form a paste. Apply this paste on your infective skin. Let it dry for 20 minutes. Wash it off with warm water. Pat dry your skin and apply some powder for drying. Repeat this process twice a day for a few days to get rid of the infection completely.

Recipe 31: Peppermint oil therapy

Peppermint is an essential oil that is believed to have a beneficial effect on skin. For treating bacterial infections, this oil is excellent. However, it should be used in diluted form to avoid its strong irritating effect on the skin.

Ingredients:

- Peppermint oil – 4 drops
- Olive oil – 2 tablespoons

Method:

Combine both the oils to make a calming ointment. With a cotton ball, apply this oil on your skin and leave it on for 20 minutes. Wash it off with warm water. This ointment doesn't only soothe your skin, but also allows flaky infective skin to come out fast so that infection disappears. Use this therapy twice a day for a few days to get instant results.

Recipe 32: Jasmine and orange oil treatment

Jasmine oil is a very effective disinfectant and antiseptic oil that can be applied to skin to cure infections. Containing Benzoic acid, Benzaldehyde and Benzyle Benzoate; this essential oil is considered highly active bactericidal, germicidal and fungicidal. Its combination with orange oil will provide calming and healing effect on your Jock Itch infection.

Ingredients:

- Jasmine oil – 4 drops
- Orange oil – 1 teaspoon

Method:

Combine both the oils to make an effective ointment. With a cotton ball, apply this oil on your skin and leave it on for 20 minutes. Wash it off with warm water. This ointment doesn't only soothe your skin, but also allows flaky infective skin to come out fast so that infection disappears. Use this therapy twice a day for a few days to get instant results.

Recipe 33: Lavender oil therapy

Oil extracted from leaves of Lavender flower is highly therapeutic and has great soothing properties that will give you respite from skin inflammation caused by infection. Also, it would allow your patchy red skin to come out in flakes that will clear the infection faster.

Ingredients:

- Lavender oil – 4 drops
- Sweet almond oil – 1 tablespoon

Method:

Mix both the oils together and apply on your skin daily, twice a day to get instant results. Also wash off the oil after 20 minutes of application and pat dry your skin to avoid moistness near the affected area.

Recipe 34: Black walnut oil treatment

Extracted from Black walnut herb, walnut oil also has strong antifungal properties that can fast cure your Jock Itch infection. It should be used in diluted form to avoid its potent effect on skin.

Ingredients:

- Black walnut oil – 1 teaspoon
- Tea Tree oil – 1 teaspoon
- Coconut oil – 1 tablespoon

Method:

Prepare a mixture of all 3 oils and apply on affected area. Leave it on for 20 minutes and wash it off with warm water. Repeat this application of oil mixture twice for a few days and see positive results.

Recipe 35: Wormwood oil application

Like other plant oils, Wormwood oil is also treated as a safe and effective oil used to cure skin diseases. When it is applied topically, it gives soothing effect on your painful rashes. Also, it helps in healing the skin to make it smooth and clean.

Ingredients:

- Wormwood oil – 1 teaspoon
- Olive oil – 1 tablespoon

Method:

Combine both the oils to make a skin ointment. Apply it on the infected skin and leave it on for 20 minutes. Wash it off and clean your skin with warm water. Repeat this treatment twice a day for a few days and you will notice the flaking of the infected skin will further clear and your infection will be healed effectively.

Part 4: Gain immunity with food!

Our body has an immune system that helps us fight against various diseases. When this immune system weakens, our body is prone to attacks from bacteria, virus and fungus. So, we must have a strong immune system to evade these deadly attacks from germs. Good food helps us gain a potent immune system. Food is an essential part of our lives that not only tickles our taste buds, but also offers health and better shape to our body. This is the reason that doctors and health experts always give stress on adopting right eating habits. In this section you can see some of the top recipes that will help you in boosting your immunity that would further assist you in avoiding fungus and bacterial attacks on your skin. Of course, every recipe has been picked up keeping in mind your taste as well!

It is instructed by doctors that starchy, sugary and fried food items may aggravate your Jock Itch condition so avoid these food items and also do not consume alcohol until your skin infection disappears. Try to include raw fruits and vegetables in your diet with lots of proteins and nuts to achieve great immunity.

Recipe 36: Apple Carrot Pear juice

To fight off infections and to have a strong immune system, our body needs Vitamin A that is available in plenty in carrots. Also the fruits and carrot boost the action of white blood cells that protects the body from attacks of foreign substances like virus, bacteria and fungus.

Ingredients:

- Carrots – 4-5 large
- Apple – 1
- Pear – 1
- Fresh ginger – $1/4^{th}$ inches

Method:

In a juicer, put all the ingredients and churn them to extract fresh juice. Pour it in glass and you can add fresh mint leaves for added flavor. Drink it twice a day to get maximum benefit. Avoid adding sugar into it.

Recipe 37: Tomato delight

You can call this juice a 'powerhouse' for immune defending properties. With the goodness of Tomato, Kale and carrots; this drink will give you immense benefits of Vitamin C, Vitamin A, Folate and Magnesium. So, better drink it twice a day to gain your immunity to fight against infections.

Ingredients:

- Tomatoes – 3
- Celery ribs – 2-3 with leaves
- Carrots – 2 medium
- Kale – 1 cup
- Sweet red bell pepper – 1
- Cilantro – 1 tablespoon
- Tabasco sauce – to taste

Method:

Put tomatoes, celery ribs, carrots, kale and bell pepper in a blender. Blend everything until smooth. Strain the puree and remove the remaining part. Pour juice in a glass, mix in Tabasco sauce and garnish with cilantro.

Recipe 38: Immune boost up Chicken Soup

Loaded with chicken proteins and antibacterial ingredients like turmeric, ginger and garlic; this soup is a power-packed entrée to enhance your immune system. Coriander added as a garnish adds anti-inflammatory and antibacterial properties to your soup, so it can be called a perfect dish to make you ready to fight against infections.

Ingredients:

- Chicken stock – 1 liter
- Chicken breast – 500 grams (cut into cubes)
- Garlic – 10 cloves (smashed)
- Ginger -2 tablespoons (finely grated)
- Fresh turmeric – 1 tablespoon (grated)
- Water – 1 liter
- Coriander – 2 bunches (chopped)
- Tamari soy sauce – 3 tablespoons
- Rice wine – ¼ cup

Method:

In a large saucepan, mix together water, stock, chicken, ginger, garlic and turmeric. Let it simmer for five to ten minutes or until chicken is fully cooked and all flavors are infused. Add wine, coriander and soy sauce. Sip slowly and enjoy!

Recipe 39: Immunity building green smoothie

Vitamin C, Zinc and Beta Carotene are some of the phytonutrients that help in building the immune system of your body. These elements also give you the strength for fighting against various germ attacks to avoid infections. So, have this smoothie twice a day to make yourself healthy with a great immune system.

Ingredients:

- Orange – 2 whole
- Lime – 1 whole
- Lemon – ½ whole
- Baby spinach leaves – a handful
- Sprig parsley – small
- Water – 1 1/2 – 2 cups (as desired)
- Watergrass juice – 1 teaspoon
- Natural immunity support powder – 1 teaspoon

Method:

Peel lemon, lime and oranges. Blend all ingredients in a blender to make smoothie. Add extra water to adjust the consistency. Pour in a tall glass and drink it to nourish yourself.

Recipe 40: Creamy mushrooms and beans

For adding flavor to your healthy food with richness of cream, you can make this green beans and mushroom dish. It's an immune boosting dish loaded with various nutrients that helps in fighting against infections.

Ingredients:

- Green beans – 450 grams (fresh or frozen) cut into 1" pieces
- Mushrooms – 450 grams (thickly sliced)
- Onion – 1/2 cup (chopped)
- Butter – 2 tablespoons
- Sour cream – ½ cup
- Black pepper – as desired, freshly ground
- Parsley – 2 tablespoons (chopped)

Method:

In a large saucepan, boil around 1 liter of water and let the beans cooked in it until tender. In a frying pan, add mushrooms and sauté until all water is dried. Remove the mushrooms from the pan and set aside. In that same frying pan, add butter and let it melt. Sauté chopped onions in butter till transparent. Now add mushrooms and beans. Fry for a minute. Lower the heat and stir in sour cream. Mix well. Sprinkle salt and pepper and mix thoroughly. Simmer for 2-3 minutes. Remove the pan from heat, transfer the mushrooms and beans into a dish and sprinkle parsley on top. Eat it with some bread and soup.

Part 5: Miscellaneous Remedies

Apart from natural oils, herbs, foods and kitchen stuff, Jock Itch can be treated using some of the surprising elements found in our household. Yes, the items that we use in our daily lives like Listerine mouthwash, nail polish, bleach, alcohol etc. have been observed to show positive results in curing rashes and skin irritation. So, why not try them to get instant relief from Jock Itch like irritating condition.

Here are methods to use certain household items for making your skin smooth and infection free.

Recipe 41: Bleach bath

Bleach bath is a good antiseptic and antifungal treatment to cure Jock Itch. It is recommended to repeat this treatment every day until you get complete relief from your infection.

Ingredients:

- Bleach – ¼ cup
- Water – a tubful

Method:

Add bleach in your bathing tub full of water and let your body soak in it for 15-20 minutes. Allow the bleach water to touch thoroughly on affected area. If your infection is severe, you can remain in the water for more minutes. Once the bath is done, pat dry your skin with a clean towel because bad hygiene and moisture can worsen the infection.

Recipe 42: Listerine mouthwash treatment

Don't get surprised to know that Listerine mouthwash can cure your skin infection. You must understand that Listerine is used to kill germs in our mouth because it contains antibacterial, antifungal and antiseptic properties. Similarly, it is able to kill the germs present on your skin specifically at the infected area. So, try it 2-3 times every day for a few months to get complete respite.

Method:

Using a cotton ball or any clean cloth, apply Listerine mouthwash on your infected skin. It may give a burning sensation initially, but you will get relief in a few minutes. Let it dry completely on its own. Your skin inflammation and soreness will disappear with continuous use and it will flake off to clear the infection.

Caution: If your have open wounds, do not use Listerine.

Recipe 43: Alcohol therapy

Doctors might say no for alcohol, but if you are suffering from Jock Itch, alcohol rub may be your best remedy. Alcohol is a fungus killer and a drying agent that will help keep your skin moisture free to avoid attack of germs.

Method:

Take 90% Isopropyl alcohol and dip a cotton ball into it. Dab the ball on your infective skin. As alcohol will vaporize easily, you are not required to wash it off. Repeat this process many times in a day until you are convinced with the results.

Recipe 44: Nail polish and nail polish remover treatment

It might be sounding really weird and hurting as well because who can think of putting nail polish remover on already infected and burning skin. But it really works!

Method:

Take a clear nail polish. Apply a single coat of nail polish on your rashes. It may give a burning sensation, but you have to bear it for a few seconds. Let the nail polish dry and remain on your skin for the entire day. In night, dip paper towel into any nail polish remover and remove the nail polish from your skin. Again, it will give extreme inflammation, but stay confident as it will give you relief in the end. When the nail polish is removed, again dip paper towel in the remover and dab on your skin. This treatment will dry your skin in a few days and your rashes will disappear.

Recipe 45: Anti-dandruff shampoo therapy

As mentioned earlier, Jock Itch is caused by the attack of fungus on the skin and similar is the case with dandruff. Hence, even an antidandruff shampoo can help treat Jock Itch successfully.

Method:

Take any antidandruff shampoo like Selsun and apply it on your affected skin. You can either use shampoo alone or dilute it with a little water. Leave it on for 10-15 minutes. Wash it off with warm water and pat dry your skin. Repeat this process daily for few months until you find it completely satisfying.

Recipe 46: Camphor therapy

Camphor has antiseptic properties that can give satisfying relief in all types of skin infections. Like it kills the yeast, a kind of fungus that causes dandruff, camphor also kills fungus that causes Jock Itch. Additionally, it gives a calming effect on your burning skin.

Ingredients:

- Camphor – 2-3
- Coconut oil – ½ cup

Method:

In a saucepan, heat oil and let camphor dissolves in it. Let it cool at room temperature. Using a cotton ball or any clean cloth, apply this oil mix on your infected skin. Leave it on for 20 minutes. Repeat this process twice a day daily until all your infection disappears.

Recipe 47: Myrrh treatment

With its effective skin healing qualities, Myrrh has been considered an ancient herbal remedy to cure skin infections and rashes. It has antiviral properties that can kill germs appeared on the skin. It is highly potent in nature, so if you have sensitive skin, avoid using it.

Ingredients:

- Myrrh oil – 1 tablespoon
- Balsam oil – 1 tablespoon

Method:

Blend both the oils and apply on your affected skin using a cotton ball. Leave it on for 20 minutes and wash it off with cold water. It will help soothe your skin and will clear your infection as well.

Recipe 48: Colloidal silver rub

Colloidal silver is a tested antibacterial cream available widely to cure all types of wounds and skin infections. It contains silver salts that help in healing skin very quickly. In Jock Itch condition, it is a very effective remedy.

Method:

Apply Colloidal silver cream generously all over your affected area and let it dry. Remove the cream using a cotton ball and wash your skin with warm water. Repeat it thrice a day for several days until your infection disappears.

Recipe 49: Green clay pack

Green clay or any healing clay makes a perfect remedy for curing skin infections. The curing properties of clay are so high that even it can treat skin cancer, which is deadly.

Ingredients:

- Green clay powder – 2-3 tablespoons
- Water – as desired to adjust the consistency
- Coconut oil – 1 teaspoon

Method:

Combine water and clay powder to make a thick paste. Pour coconut oil in it and mix. Apply this pack to your affected skin and let it dry for 1-2 hours. Wash it off with warm water and pat dry your skin. Repeat this process daily for fast results.

Recipe 50: Petroleum Jelly treatment

Petroleum jelly is a very effective remedy to soften your skin tremendously. It has antiseptic properties that work well on your skin.

Method:

Apply petroleum jelly all over your affected skin and leave it on for 15 minutes. Remove it with a cotton ball and wash it off with warm water. Repeat it thrice a day for a few days to get instant results.

Conclusion

By now you must have understood that Jock Itch is a condition that aggravates with moisture, so you are advised to keep your affected area like groin and inner thighs completely dry. Whichever home remedy you apply, you must take care of personal hygiene and daily activities to avoid unnecessary stress on your infected skin.

With a hectic life, when you cannot sit at home all day, especially if you are working or are an active person, you must see to it that most of your time at home should be relaxing. Also adopt activities that do not generally heighten your infection.

Here we also want to stress on taking measures to keep your body hygienic because fungus and bacteria like germs usually attack on dirty skin. However, if by chance, you are suffering from a skin infection, then make sure that your personal belongings like soap, tooth brush, towel and clothes are kept separately. Also, wash your clothes separately as Jock Itch and other skin infections are contagious. Use a mild antiseptic detergent to wash your clothes and other belongings. Specifically, you should avoid close contact with kids because baby skin is more prone to catch skin infections.

Along with our recommended home remedies, you also take care that you do not unnecessarily scratch your rashes. This practice will maximize your skin ailment, rather than giving you relief.

So, now when you are aware of top 50 home remedial methods to cure your Jock Itch infection, your infection will not last longer. If you follow the steps given in the recipes, you will be able to evade this irritating infection successfully. However, we never say no to medications that are available over the counter or with prescription as these medicines and ointments will definitely help along with these home remedies.

Our book is a comprehensive guide for you and we advise you to read it whenever you have any Jock like condition. We thank you for downloading this book and encourage us to write more such book for our patrons. If you really like the content and your skin infection is relieved from any of our home remedies, then kindly take your time to write a feedback in our comments section. Your views are valuable for us and for new readers. Till the happy healing!

ABOUT THE AUTHOR

Rita Clark is an author of natural remedies, herbal remedies, and medicine books, ranking among the top 30 most popular authors in Health, Fitness & Dieting plus Alternative Medicine on Amazon AuthorRank.

Rita's experience includes 15 years in the herbal community as a healer, teacher, visionary, and organizer of herbal events.

Currently, Rita resides in the San Francisco Bay Area with her family, Whiskey. She enjoys teaching, planting trees, and going on vacation when she has free time.

Feel Free to contact me via ritaclarkrecipes@gmail.com

Made in the USA
Monee, IL
21 June 2021